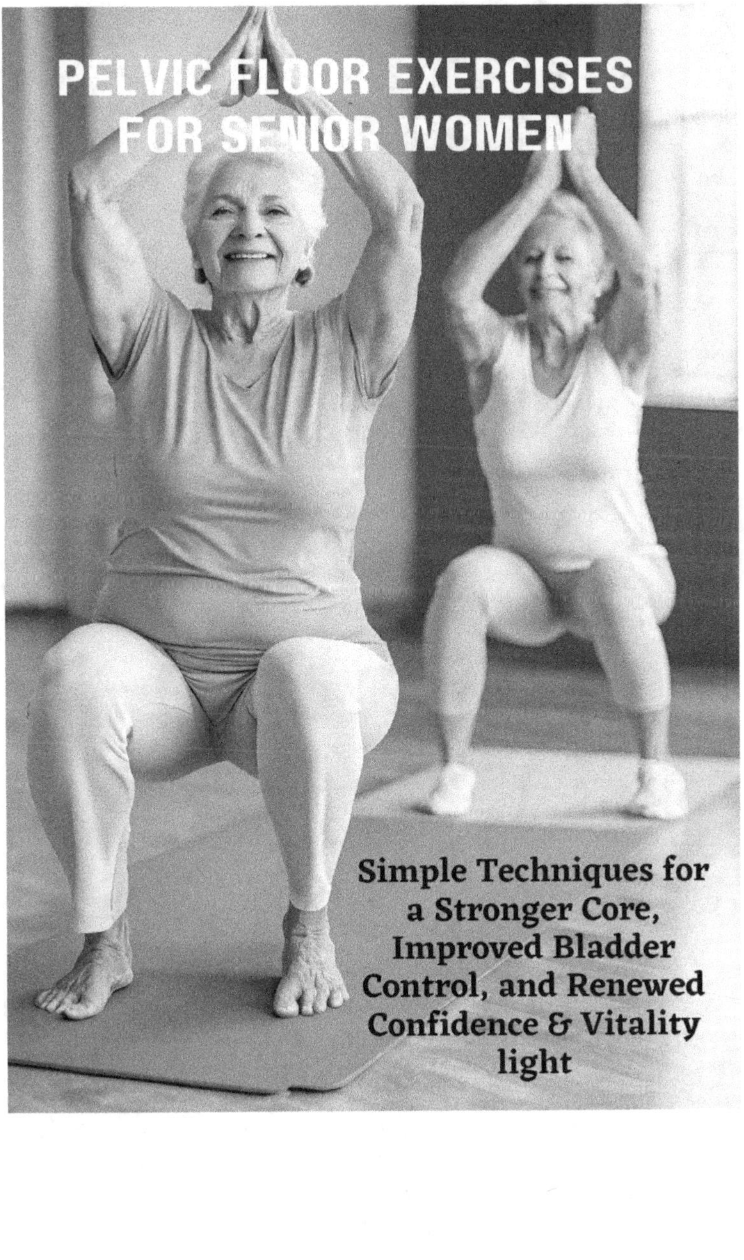

# PELVIC FLOOR EXERCISES FOR SENIOR WOMEN

## Simple Techniques for a Stronger Core, Improved Bladder Control, and Renewed Confidence & Vitality

light

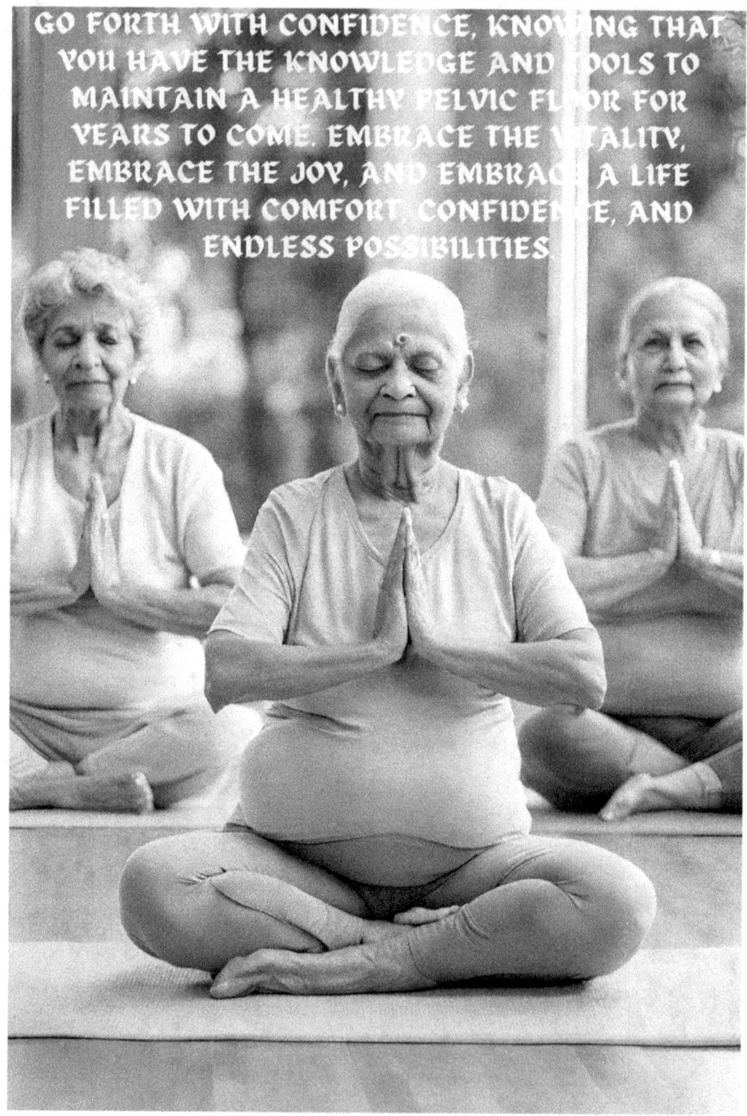

GO FORTH WITH CONFIDENCE, KNOWING THAT YOU HAVE THE KNOWLEDGE AND TOOLS TO MAINTAIN A HEALTHY PELVIC FLOOR FOR YEARS TO COME. EMBRACE THE VITALITY, EMBRACE THE JOY, AND EMBRACE A LIFE FILLED WITH COMFORT, CONFIDENCE, AND ENDLESS POSSIBILITIES.

Remember, you are not alone. Millions of women are on this journey with you, seeking to improve their pelvic health and quality of life. Together, we can break down barriers, shatter stigmas, and empower women to take charge of their well-being.

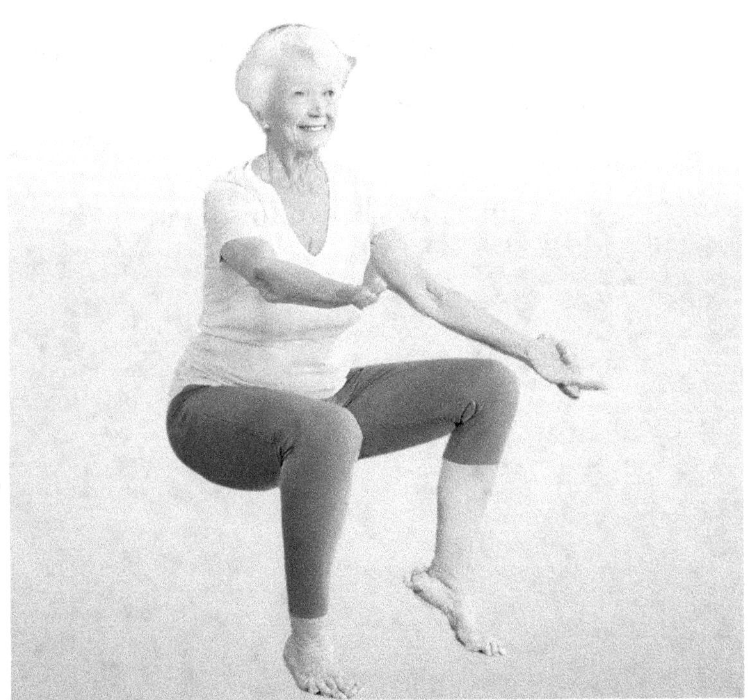

# TABLE OF CONTENTS

# INTRODUCTION

## REDISCOVERING YOUR VITALITY

### A JOURNEY TO STRENGTH AND CONFIDENCE

Welcome to a new chapter in your life—a chapter where you reclaim your strength, vitality, and confidence, all from the comfort of your own home.

If you're a senior woman seeking a safe, effective, and empowering way to enhance your well-being, you've come to the right place. This book is your guide to unlocking the transformative power of pelvic floor exercises, designed specifically for you.

Now, you might be wondering, "What exactly are pelvic floor exercises, and why should I care?" Well, let's dive into that. Your pelvic floor is a group of muscles, ligaments, and tissues that form a supportive hammock at the base of your pelvis.

These muscles play a crucial role in bladder and bowel control, core stability, and even sexual function. However, as we age, these muscles can weaken due to various factors, including childbirth, hormonal changes, and the natural aging process.

The good news is that pelvic floor exercises, sometimes called Kegels, can significantly improve the strength and function of these muscles. Think of it like giving your body's foundation a much-needed tune-up.

By regularly practicing these simple yet powerful exercises, you can experience a wide range of benefits, including:

- **Improved Bladder Control**

Regain confidence and peace of mind by reducing or eliminating leaks and the urgency to go.

- **Enhanced Core Strength**

Strengthen your core muscles for better balance, posture, and overall stability.

- **Increased Vitality**

Feel more energized and vibrant as you improve your pelvic floor health.

- **Boosted Confidence**

Reclaim your sense of self-assurance and enjoy activities without

- **Reduced Pain and Discomfort**

Alleviate pelvic pain and discomfort for a more comfortable and enjoyable life.

- **Improved Sexual Function**

Enhance your sexual health and satisfaction.

You might be thinking, "But I'm not a fitness enthusiast. Are these exercises safe and easy for me?" Absolutely! Pelvic floor exercises are gentle, low-impact, and adaptable to your fitness level and individual needs.

This book will guide you through each step, ensuring that you practice safely and effectively.

We'll dispel common myths and misconceptions about pelvic floor health, address concerns you may have, and provide clear instructions with modifications for different abilities.

What sets this book apart is its focus on you, the senior woman. We understand the unique challenges and concerns you may face as you age. That's why we've created a program that is accessible, empowering, and tailored to your specific needs. We'll celebrate your strengths, encourage your progress, and provide a supportive community to share your journey.

This book is not just about exercises; it's about embracing a healthier, more vibrant life. We'll delve into lifestyle tips, nutrition, and other holistic practices that can further enhance your pelvic floor health and overall well-being. You'll discover inspiring stories from other senior women who have transformed their lives through pelvic floor fitness. Their journeys will motivate and encourage you as you embark on your own path to renewed vitality.

So, take a deep breath, relax your shoulders, and get ready to discover the incredible potential of your pelvic floor. This book is your invitation to rediscover your inner strength, regain your confidence, and embrace a life filled with comfort, vitality, and joy. Let's embark on this empowering journey together!

# CHAPTER ONE

## AWAKENING YOUR INNER STRENGTH: THE POWER OF THE PELVIC FLOOR

### WHY PELVIC HEALTH MATTERS FOR SENIOR WOMEN

Let's talk about something that affects millions of women, yet is rarely discussed openly: pelvic floor health. It's a topic often shrouded in secrecy and embarrassment, but it's time to shed light on this vital aspect of well-being, especially for senior women.

The pelvic floor, a group of muscles, ligaments, and tissues at the base of your pelvis, is your body's unsung hero. It supports your bladder, uterus, and bowel, and it plays a crucial role in bladder and bowel control, sexual function, and even core stability. However, as we age, these muscles can weaken due to childbirth, hormonal changes, menopause, and other factors.

The statistics are eye-opening: studies show that up to 50% of women experience some form of pelvic floor dysfunction in their lifetime. For senior women, the numbers are even higher, with some estimates suggesting that over 70% experience symptoms like urinary incontinence, pelvic organ prolapse, or bowel problems. These issues can significantly impact your quality of life, leading to physical discomfort, emotional distress, and social isolation.

Imagine the frustration of constantly worrying about leaks or accidents, the embarrassment of having to plan your outings around bathroom breaks, or the fear of engaging in activities you once enjoyed. These are just some of the emotional burdens that pelvic floor problems can bring.

But it doesn't have to be this way. The good news is that pelvic floor issues are often treatable, and in many cases, preventable. By understanding the importance of pelvic health and taking proactive steps to strengthen your pelvic floor muscles, you can regain control, confidence, and a renewed sense of vitality.

It's time to break the silence surrounding pelvic health. Talking openly about these issues is the first step towards finding solutions and support. Share your experiences with friends, family, or healthcare providers. You'll be surprised to learn how many women are facing similar challenges and are eager to find relief.

Remember, you are not alone in this journey. There are countless resources available to help you, from informative books like this one to qualified healthcare professionals who specialize in pelvic floor therapy. Don't hesitate to seek guidance and support from those who can help you understand your options and develop a personalized plan to address your specific needs.

By prioritizing your pelvic health, you're investing in your overall well-being. Strong pelvic floor muscles can improve your posture, enhance your core strength, and boost your energy levels. You'll feel more confident and empowered to engage in activities you love, whether it's dancing, gardening, or simply enjoying time with loved ones.

So, let's embark on this journey together. Let's unravel the mysteries of the pelvic floor, dispel the myths, and embrace the power of knowledge and self-care. It's time to reclaim your comfort, your confidence, and your vitality. Your pelvic health matters, and it's never too late to take charge of it.

## BEYOND KEGELS: THE MULTIFACETED BENEFITS OF PELVIC FLOOR FITNESS

Imagine a life where you feel confident, comfortable, and in control of your body. A life where you can laugh freely, sneeze without worry, and enjoy your favorite activities without a second thought. These might seem like simple pleasures, but for many women, they can become distant dreams due to pelvic floor weakness. Fortunately, there's a path to reclaim that control and vitality: pelvic floor fitness.

While Kegel exercises are a well-known starting point, the benefits of a strong pelvic floor extend far beyond improved bladder control. Think of your pelvic floor as the foundation of your core – a network of muscles that support your bladder, uterus, bowel, and lower back.

When these muscles are strong, they provide a solid base for your entire body, leading to improved posture and reduced strain on your spine. This can alleviate back pain, enhance your balance and coordination, and even make everyday movements feel more effortless.

Imagine walking taller, sitting straighter, and moving with a newfound grace and ease. These are just some of the transformative effects that pelvic floor fitness can have on your physical well-being.

But the benefits don't stop there. A strong pelvic floor is also intimately connected to your sexual health and satisfaction. Pelvic floor muscles play a key role in arousal, orgasm, and overall sexual function.

By strengthening these muscles, you can experience heightened sensitivity, increased pleasure, and even a boost in libido. It's a natural and empowering way to reignite the spark in your intimate life.

Moreover, pelvic floor fitness can have a profound impact on your emotional and mental well-being. The confidence that comes with improved bladder control and reduced discomfort can lift your spirits and enhance your self-esteem. You'll feel more at ease in social situations, knowing that you're not limited by worries about leaks or accidents. This newfound freedom can lead to increased social engagement, a more active lifestyle, and a greater sense of overall happiness.

Think of pelvic floor fitness as a holistic approach to well-being. It's not just about preventing leaks or improving bladder control; it's about unlocking a cascade of positive effects that ripple through every aspect of your life. By strengthening your pelvic floor, you're strengthening your body, your mind, and your spirit.

It's important to remember that pelvic floor fitness is a journey, not a destination. It takes time, dedication, and the right guidance to achieve optimal results. But with the right exercises, techniques, and support, you can experience a profound transformation in your health and well-being.

So, let's go beyond Kegels and explore the full spectrum of benefits that pelvic floor fitness has to offer. Let's embrace a holistic approach to strengthening your core, boosting your confidence, and reclaiming your vitality. Your road to a happy, healthier self starts today.

# CHAPTER TWO

## DEMYSTIFYING THE PELVIC FLOOR: YOUR FOUNDATION FOR VITALITY

### UNDERSTANDING YOUR BODY'S HIDDEN GEM

Think of your body as a beautifully designed house, with each room serving a specific purpose. Your core, the central part of your body, is the foundation upon which this house stands. And within this core lies a hidden gem, a group of muscles that often go unnoticed but play a vital role in your overall health and well-being: your pelvic floor.

Imagine your pelvic floor as a hammock of muscles, ligaments, and tissues that stretches across the base of your pelvis. It's like a supportive sling that cradles your bladder, uterus, and bowel, keeping them in their proper positions and functioning optimally. This intricate network of muscles is responsible for several essential functions:

- ### Bladder and Bowel Control

Your pelvic floor muscles act as gatekeepers, controlling the flow of urine and stool. When these muscles contract, they close the openings of your bladder and rectum, preventing leaks and accidents. When they relax, they allow for normal emptying.

- ### Core Stability

Your pelvic floor muscles are part of your core, a group of muscles that work together to stabilize your spine and pelvis. A strong pelvic floor contributes to good posture, balance, and coordination. It helps support your back, reducing the risk of pain and injury.

- ### Sexual Function

Your pelvic floor muscles are intimately connected to your sexual health. During arousal and orgasm, these muscles contract and relax rhythmically, enhancing sensation and pleasure. A strong pelvic floor can contribute to a more satisfying sex life.

- **Organ Support**

As we age, the pelvic floor muscles can weaken, leading to issues like pelvic organ prolapse, where one or more of the pelvic organs (bladder, uterus, or rectum) can drop down from their normal position. Strong pelvic floor muscles help to keep these organs in place, preventing discomfort and dysfunction.

Let's take a closer look at the structure of your pelvic floor. Imagine three layers of muscles stacked on top of each other, forming a supportive bowl-like shape. The deepest layer, closest to your spine, consists of muscles that run from the front to the back of your pelvis, forming a supportive sling.

The middle layer is made up of muscles that wrap around your openings, helping to control bladder and bowel function. The outermost layer includes muscles that surround the opening of your vagina and anus.

Understanding the anatomy of your pelvic floor can empower you to take charge of your health. By visualizing these muscles and their functions, you can better connect with them and appreciate their importance.

Now, you might be wondering, "What does my pelvic floor look like?" Well, it's not something you can see from the outside, but you can certainly feel it. Imagine squeezing the muscles you would use to stop the flow of urine or prevent passing gas. Your pelvic floor muscles are in action there!

Take a moment to connect with these muscles right now. Gently squeeze them, hold for a few seconds, and then release. Notice the sensation of lifting and tightening as you contract, and the feeling of relaxation as you let go. This simple exercise is a great way to start building awareness and strength in your pelvic floor.

## RECOGNIZING THE CHALLENGES OF AGING AND PELVIC HEALTH

Just as our skin wrinkles and our bones may become less dense over time, the muscles of our pelvic floor also undergo changes as we age. While aging is a natural and beautiful process, it's important to understand how it can affect our pelvic health so we can take proactive steps to maintain strength and vitality.

Think of your pelvic floor muscles like any other muscle in your body. They thrive on regular use and exercise, but they can weaken and lose tone if neglected. Several factors contribute to this decline in pelvic floor function, especially as we enter our senior years.

Childbirth, for instance, can stretch and strain the pelvic floor muscles, especially during vaginal deliveries. While many women regain strength in these muscles postpartum, some may experience lingering weakness that can worsen with age.

Menopause is another significant factor. As estrogen levels decline, the tissues of the pelvic floor can become thinner and less elastic, making them more prone to weakness and injury.

But childbirth and menopause are not the only culprits. Other age-related changes, such as decreased muscle mass and reduced nerve function, can also contribute to pelvic floor weakness. Chronic conditions like diabetes, obesity, and chronic obstructive pulmonary disease (COPD) can further exacerbate the problem.

Lifestyle factors also play a role. A sedentary lifestyle, chronic constipation, and repetitive heavy lifting can put excessive strain on the pelvic floor muscles, leading to weakness over time. Additionally, certain medications, such as diuretics and antihistamines, can contribute to bladder problems and pelvic floor dysfunction.

It is noteworthy that the experiences of individual women are not the same. Some women may sail through menopause with minimal pelvic floor issues, while others may experience significant changes. The good news is that regardless of your individual circumstances, there are steps you can take to protect and strengthen your pelvic floor at any age.

Understanding the factors that contribute to pelvic floor weakness is the first step towards taking control of your health. By recognizing the potential challenges, you can make informed decisions about your lifestyle, seek appropriate guidance from healthcare professionals, and implement strategies to maintain a strong and healthy pelvic floor.

Knowledge is power. By educating yourself about the changes that occur in your body as you age, you can take proactive steps to prevent or manage pelvic floor problems. This might involve making simple lifestyle modifications, such as maintaining a healthy weight, staying active, and practicing good bowel habits. It may also involve seeking professional guidance from a pelvic floor therapist or other healthcare provider who can assess your specific needs and recommend a personalized treatment plan.

Remember, you are not alone in this journey. Millions of women experience pelvic floor issues, and there are a wealth of resources available to support you. By breaking the silence and seeking help, you can overcome these challenges and embrace a life of confidence, comfort, and vitality.

# CHAPTER THREE

## YOUR PELVIC FLOOR FITNESS JOURNEY BEGINS: GENTLE FIRST STEPS

### SIMPLE TECHNIQUES TO CONNECT WITH YOUR PELVIC FLOOR - FINDING YOUR FOUNDATION

Ready to embark on your pelvic floor fitness journey? Let's begin with the most fundamental step: getting acquainted with your pelvic floor muscles. Like any good relationship, this one starts with understanding and connection. It's easier than you would imagine, which is fantastic news!

**Picture this:** your pelvic floor muscles are like a sling or hammock that stretches across the base of your pelvis. They support your bladder, uterus, and bowel. To connect with them, imagine you're trying to stop the flow of urine midstream or prevent passing gas. That squeezing sensation you feel? That's your pelvic floor muscles contracting.

Now, let's try a few gentle exercises to isolate and strengthen these muscles. Choose a comfortable posture to lie in, sit in, or stand in. Relax your body, especially your belly, thighs, and buttocks. Breathe deeply in and out for a few moments, releasing any tension.

**The Elevator:** Imagine your pelvic floor is an elevator with several floors. Slowly contract your muscles as if you're lifting the elevator from the ground floor to the first floor. Hold the contraction for a few seconds, then slowly release, lowering the elevator back down. Repeat this several times, gradually increasing the number of "floors" as you get stronger.

**The Bridge:** Lie on your back with your knees bent and feet flat on the floor. Gently engage your pelvic floor muscles as if you're lifting them up and in. At the same time, lift your hips off the floor, creating a straight line from your knees to your shoulders. After a little period of holding, gradually bring your hips back down. Keep in mind to breathe normally while performing the activity.

**The Squeeze and Release:** This is the classic Kegel exercise. Simply squeeze your pelvic floor muscles as if you're stopping the flow of urine, hold for a few seconds, and then release. Repeat this several times. You can do Kegels anytime, anywhere – while sitting at your desk, watching TV, or even waiting in line at the grocery store.

As you practice these exercises, focus on feeling the contraction and release of your pelvic floor muscles. Avoid clenching your buttocks, thighs, or abdominal muscles. If you're unsure whether you're doing it correctly, place your fingers on your perineum (the area between your vagina and anus). You should feel a gentle lift and squeeze as you contract your pelvic floor muscles.

Remember, consistency is key! Aim to do these exercises several times a day, gradually increasing the number of repetitions and hold time as you get stronger. It's crucial to pay attention to your body's signals and stop if you experience any pain or discomfort.

If you're new to pelvic floor exercises, it's a good idea to start with the guidance of a pelvic floor therapist or other healthcare provider. They can assess your individual needs and recommend a personalized exercise program that's safe and effective for you.

With practice and patience, you'll develop a stronger connection with your pelvic floor muscles and reap the many benefits of pelvic floor fitness. So, take a deep breath, relax, and start exploring this hidden gem within your body. Your journey to improved health and well-being begins now.

## POWER OF BREATH FOR SUPPORT - BREATHING LIFE INTO YOUR PELVIS

Did you know that something as simple and natural as your breath can have a profound impact on your pelvic floor health? It's true! Your breath and your pelvic floor are like dance partners, moving in sync with each other. When your breath is shallow and restricted, your pelvic floor muscles tend to tense up, while deep, diaphragmatic breathing promotes relaxation and support.

Imagine your diaphragm, the large dome-shaped muscle that sits below your lungs, as the top of a balloon. Your pelvic floor muscles form the bottom of this balloon. When you inhale deeply, your diaphragm contracts and moves downward, gently pushing your abdominal organs down and outward. This creates space for your pelvic floor muscles to lengthen and relax. When you exhale, your diaphragm relaxes and rises, allowing your pelvic floor muscles to gently lift and contract.

This coordinated movement, like a gentle massage, is essential for maintaining a healthy and supple pelvic floor. When we breathe shallowly, using primarily our chest muscles, we miss out on this natural movement. This can lead to chronic tension in the pelvic floor, contributing to issues like incontinence, pelvic pain, and even sexual dysfunction.

Diaphragmatic breathing, also known as belly breathing, is a simple yet powerful technique that can help you restore this natural rhythm and promote optimal pelvic floor function. To practice diaphragmatic breathing, find a comfortable position, either lying down or sitting with your back straight. Place one hand to your stomach and another to your chest. As you inhale slowly and deeply through your nose, feel your belly rise while your chest remains relatively still. Exhale slowly through your mouth, feeling your belly fall.

As you practice this breathing technique, visualize your pelvic floor muscles expanding and relaxing with each inhale and gently lifting and contracting with each exhale. With regular practice, diaphragmatic breathing can become second nature, benefiting your pelvic floor health and overall well-being.

Beyond diaphragmatic breathing, there are other breathing exercises you can explore to further enhance pelvic floor function. For example, try "breath holds," where you inhale deeply, hold your breath for a few seconds, and then exhale slowly. This can help strengthen your pelvic floor muscles and improve their coordination.

Another helpful exercise is "reverse breathing," where you inhale and gently contract your pelvic floor muscles, then exhale and relax them. This exercise can be particularly beneficial for women experiencing pelvic floor tightness or pain.

Also Remember, the key is to breathe deeply and fully, allowing your diaphragm to move freely and your pelvic floor muscles to respond naturally. As you practice these exercises, pay attention to your body's signals and adjust your breath as needed. Stop and speak with a healthcare provider if you feel any discomfort.

Breathing exercises are a gentle and accessible way to nurture your pelvic floor health. By incorporating them into your daily routine, you can improve bladder and bowel control, reduce pain and discomfort, enhance sexual function, and even boost your energy levels and mood. So, take a deep breath and discover the transformative power of your breath for a healthier, happier you.

# CHAPTER FOUR

## BUILDING A STRONGER CORE: ESSENTIAL EXERCISES FOR EVERYDAY CONFIDENCE

## KEGELS DEMYSTIFIED: MASTERING THE BASICS FOR A STRONGER FOUNDATION

Ready to unlock the secret to a stronger, more resilient pelvic floor? Kegel exercises, often hailed as the cornerstone of pelvic floor fitness, are a simple yet powerful tool for improving bladder control, enhancing core strength, and revitalizing your overall well-being. Let's demystify this essential practice and guide you through the proper techniques for optimal results.

At their core, Kegel exercises involve contracting and relaxing the muscles of your pelvic floor. Imagine the feeling of stopping the flow of urine midstream or preventing passing gas. That's what it feels like to engage your pelvic floor muscles. But it's not just about squeezing; it's about doing it correctly to maximize the benefits and avoid straining other muscles.

Here is a detailed outline on how to complete Kegel exercises:

- **Find Your Muscles**

Begin by identifying your pelvic floor muscles. The easiest way to do this is to stop the flow of urine while you're using the bathroom. Once you've located the muscles, you can practice contracting and relaxing them without actually stopping your urine flow.

- **Get Comfortable**

Find a comfortable position, either lying down, sitting, or standing. Relax your body, especially your abdomen, thighs, and buttocks.

- **Squeeze and Lift**

Gently squeeze your pelvic floor muscles as if you're lifting them up and in. Imagine drawing your muscles up towards your belly button. Hold the contraction for 3-5 seconds, then slowly release.

- **Focus on Isolation**

As you contract your pelvic floor muscles, avoid squeezing your buttocks, thighs, or abdominal muscles. Breathe normally throughout the exercise.

- **Repeat and Progress**

Start with 10 repetitions, holding each contraction for 3-5 seconds. As you gain strength, progressively lengthen the holds. Every day, try to perform three sets of ten repetitions.

Now that you've mastered the basic Kegel, let's explore some variations to keep your routine engaging and challenge your muscles further:

- **Quick Flicks**

Instead of holding the contraction, quickly squeeze and release your pelvic floor muscles several times in a row.

- **The Elevator**

Imagine your pelvic floor is an elevator with several floors. Slowly contract your muscles as if you're lifting the elevator from the ground floor to the first floor, then the second, and so on. Hold each contraction for a few seconds, then slowly release, lowering the elevator back down.

- **Long Holds**

Challenge yourself to hold a Kegel contraction for as long as you can, gradually increasing the time as you get stronger. Aim for 10 seconds or more.

Remember, consistency is key. Incorporate Kegel exercises into your daily routine, whether you're watching TV, reading a book, or even brushing your teeth. With regular practice, you'll notice a significant improvement in your pelvic floor strength and function.

If you're unsure whether you're performing Kegel exercises correctly, don't hesitate to seek guidance from a pelvic floor therapist or other healthcare provider. They can provide personalized instruction and feedback to ensure you're getting the most out of your exercises.

## GENTLE MOVEMENTS, POWERFUL IMPACT: INCORPORATING PELVIC FLOOR EXERCISE INTO DAILY LIFE

Incorporating pelvic floor exercises into your daily life doesn't require a trip to the gym or a dedicated workout session. In fact, some of the most effective exercises can be seamlessly woven into your everyday routines, making it easy to prioritize your pelvic health without disrupting your schedule. Here's how you can strengthen your pelvic floor while going about your day:

- **Sitting Pretty: Pelvic Floor Engagement at Your Desk**

The next time you're sitting at your desk, answering emails, or balancing your checkbook, take a moment to engage your pelvic floor muscles. Simply squeeze and lift your muscles as if you're trying to stop the flow of urine. For a few seconds, hold the contraction, then release. Repeat this several times throughout the day. This discreet exercise is a great way to work your pelvic floor while staying productive.

- **Standing Tall: Pelvic Floor Activation While Waiting**

Whether you're waiting in line at the grocery store, standing at the sink washing dishes, or waiting for the bus, you can subtly engage your pelvic floor muscles. Imagine drawing your muscles up and in, as if you're pulling them towards your belly button.For a few seconds, hold the contraction, then release. This simple exercise not only strengthens your pelvic floor but also improves your posture and core stability.

- **Chore Time Workout: Pelvic Floor Fitness During Household Tasks**

Transform your household chores into a workout for your pelvic floor. As you're folding laundry, vacuuming, or sweeping the floor, practice Kegel exercises or quick flicks (rapid contractions and releases). You can also try engaging your pelvic floor muscles while you're lifting or carrying objects, as this helps to support your lower back and prevent strain.

- **Mindful Moments: Pelvic Floor Awareness Throughout the Day**

Cultivate awareness of your pelvic floor muscles throughout the day. Pay attention to how they feel when you're sitting, standing, walking, or even laughing or coughing. Notice any tension or weakness, and gently engage the muscles to provide support and stability. This mindful approach can help you identify triggers for pelvic floor dysfunction and develop strategies to prevent leaks or discomfort.

- **Breathing and Movement Integration: Yoga and Pilates for Pelvic Health**

Consider incorporating gentle movement practices like yoga or Pilates into your routine. These disciplines often include exercises that specifically target the pelvic floor, such as bridge pose, cat-cow pose, and pelvic tilts. They also emphasize deep breathing, which, as we've discussed, is essential for pelvic floor relaxation and function.

By integrating these simple exercises and techniques into your daily life, you'll be surprised at how quickly you can strengthen your pelvic floor and improve your overall well-being. Remember, consistency is key. The more you practice, the stronger and more resilient your pelvic floor muscles will become.

It's crucial to pay attention to your body and modify the workouts as necessary. In the event that you feel any pain or discomfort, stop and seek medical advice. They can help you modify the exercises or recommend alternative approaches that are safe and effective for you.

So, embrace the power of movement and make pelvic floor fitness a natural part of your daily life.

By doing so, you'll not only improve your pelvic health but also enhance your overall quality of life

# CHAPTER FIVE

## EMBRACING A VIBRANT LIFE: ELEVATING YOUR PELVIC FLOOR FITNESS

## BEYOND THE BASICS: EXPLORING INTERMEDIATE AND ADVANCED TECHNIQUES

Congratulations! You've mastered the basics of pelvic floor exercise and are ready to take your fitness to the next level. Just like any muscle group, your pelvic floor thrives on challenge and variety. Let's explore some intermediate and advanced techniques that will not only strengthen your pelvic floor but also enhance your overall well-being.

First on our list is the reverse Kegel. While Kegels focus on contracting your pelvic floor muscles, reverse Kegels involve the opposite action: relaxation. This exercise is crucial for maintaining a healthy balance between contraction and relaxation, preventing muscle tightness and improving pelvic floor flexibility. To perform a reverse Kegel, simply imagine letting go of your pelvic floor muscles completely, as if you're allowing urine to flow. Hold the relaxation for a few seconds, then gently contract your muscles back up. Repeat this several times.

Next up, let's revisit the elevator exercise, but with a twist. Instead of just going up and down, imagine your pelvic floor elevator has multiple stops between floors. Slowly contract your muscles, stopping at each imaginary floor along the way. Hold each contraction for a few seconds before moving up to the next floor. Then, slowly release your muscles, stopping at each floor on the way down. This variation helps to train your pelvic floor muscles to contract and relax with greater control and precision.

Now, let's stretch things out. Pelvic floor stretches are often overlooked, but they are essential for maintaining flexibility and preventing tightness.

One simple stretch is the Happy Baby pose. Lie on your back, bend your knees towards your chest, and grab the outsides of your feet with your hands. Gently pull your knees towards your armpits, feeling a stretch in your pelvic floor muscles. Hold for 15-30 seconds, breathing deeply.

Another effective stretch is the Child's Pose. Place your big toes together while kneeling on the ground. Sit back on your heels and fold your torso over your thighs, reaching your arms out in front of you. Relax your pelvic floor muscles and allow your belly to rest on your thighs. Hold for 30-60 seconds, breathing deeply.

As you progress in your pelvic floor fitness journey, you can explore other advanced techniques, such as:

- **The Knack**

This involves contracting your pelvic floor muscles just before and during activities that put pressure on your bladder, such as coughing, sneezing, or lifting.

- **Hypopressives**

These are specialized breathing exercises that involve creating a vacuum-like effect in your abdomen, which can help to lift and support your pelvic organs.

Remember, these are just a few examples of the many exercises and techniques available to strengthen and tone your pelvic floor. Finding a routine that suits your body and yourself is important. If you're unsure where to start, or if you have any concerns about pelvic floor dysfunction, don't hesitate to seek guidance from a pelvic floor therapist or other healthcare provider.

By challenging your pelvic floor muscles with a variety of exercises, you can achieve optimal strength, flexibility, and function. This will not only improve your bladder control and core stability but also enhance your overall well-being, allowing you to live life with confidence, comfort, and vitality.

## RECLAIMING INTIMACY: NURTURING YOUR PELVIC FLOOR FOR A FULFILLING LIFE

Intimacy is a beautiful and essential part of life, enriching our relationships and nourishing our souls. For many women, however, physical and emotional changes associated with aging can create challenges in the realm of intimacy. The good news is that pelvic floor health plays a pivotal role in sexual function and satisfaction, and with the right knowledge and care, you can reclaim your confidence and pleasure.

Your pelvic floor muscles are not just about bladder control and core stability; they are also intimately connected to your sexual well-being. These muscles surround and support your vagina, clitoris, and other pelvic organs, contributing to arousal, sensation, and orgasm.

A strong pelvic floor can enhance sensitivity during intimacy, allowing you to experience heightened pleasure and deeper orgasms. It can also improve vaginal lubrication and tightness, contributing to greater comfort and satisfaction for both you and your partner.

On the other hand, a weak pelvic floor can lead to a range of issues that can impact your intimate life. Decreased sensitivity, difficulty achieving orgasm, and painful intercourse are just a few of the challenges that can arise. Pelvic organ prolapse, a condition where one or more pelvic organs drop from their normal position, can also cause discomfort and interfere with sexual activity.

But there's hope! By prioritizing your pelvic floor health, you can address these issues and reclaim your intimate life. Pelvic floor exercises, such as Kegels and other techniques we've discussed, can significantly improve muscle tone and function.

Here are some specific tips and exercises to enhance intimacy and pleasure:

- **Kegel Variations**

Explore different Kegel variations, such as quick flicks and the elevator exercise, to challenge and strengthen your pelvic floor muscles.

- **Pelvic Floor Stretches**

Gentle stretches like Happy Baby pose and Child's Pose can help to relax and lengthen your pelvic floor muscles, promoting flexibility and reducing tension.

- **Mindful Intimacy**

During intimacy, focus on connecting with your pelvic floor muscles. Notice how they contract and relax as you become aroused. Experiment with consciously engaging and releasing these muscles to enhance sensation and pleasure.

- **Communication with Your Partner**

Open and honest communication with your partner is key to a fulfilling intimate life. Share your needs and concerns, and work together to find positions and techniques that feel comfortable and pleasurable for both of you.

Never forget that intimacy is about more than just physical pleasure. It's about emotional connection, trust, and vulnerability. By nurturing your pelvic floor health, you're not only improving your physical function but also fostering a deeper sense of well-being and confidence that can positively impact your relationships and overall quality of life.

If you're experiencing any pain or discomfort during intimacy, or if you have concerns about your pelvic floor health, don't hesitate to seek guidance from a healthcare provider. They can help you address any underlying issues and develop a personalized plan to enhance your sexual well-being.

So, embrace the power of pelvic floor fitness and reclaim your intimacy. With dedication, patience, and the right guidance, you can rediscover the joy and pleasure that intimacy brings, enhancing your relationships and overall well-being.

# CHAPTER SIX

## NOURISHING YOUR PELVIC FLOOR: LIFESTYLE TIPS FOR LIFELONG HEALTH

### NUTRITION: FOODS AND SUPPLEMENTS TO SUPPORT PELVIC HEALTH

You've likely heard the saying, "You are what you eat." When it comes to pelvic health, this adage rings especially true. The foods you choose to nourish your body can significantly impact the strength and function of your pelvic floor muscles. A balanced diet rich in essential nutrients not only supports overall health but also plays a crucial role in maintaining a healthy pelvic floor.

Let's explore the nutritional building blocks that can bolster your pelvic floor fitness journey:

- **Fiber: Your Pelvic Floor's Best Friend**

Fiber is essential for maintaining healthy bowel movements and preventing constipation, which can strain your pelvic floor muscles. Aim to include plenty of high-fiber foods in your diet, such as fruits, vegetables, whole grains, and legumes. Think of vibrant berries, crunchy carrots, hearty whole-wheat bread, and satisfying lentil soup. These foods not only support your pelvic floor but also provide a wealth of other health benefits, including improved digestion and reduced risk of chronic diseases.

- **Hydration: The Elixir of Pelvic Health**

Water is essential for all bodily functions, including pelvic floor health. Staying hydrated helps to keep your tissues lubricated and supple, promoting optimal muscle function and reducing the risk of constipation. Aim to drink plenty of water throughout the day, and consider adding herbal teas or infused water for a flavorful twist. If you have any concerns about your fluid intake, consult your healthcare provider for personalized recommendations.

- **Protein: The Building Blocks of Strong Muscles**

Your pelvic floor muscles, like any other muscles in your body, need protein to stay strong and healthy. Include good sources of protein in your diet, such as lean meats, fish, poultry, beans, lentils, tofu, and dairy products. These foods provide the amino acids necessary for muscle repair and growth, ensuring your pelvic floor stays in tip-top shape.

- **Magnesium: The Relaxation Mineral**

One mineral that is essential for relaxing muscles is magnesium. Adequate magnesium intake can help to prevent muscle cramps and spasms, which can sometimes affect the pelvic floor. Take foods high in magnesium, such as legumes, whole grains, nuts, and seeds, as well as leafy green vegetables. If you're concerned about your magnesium levels, talk to your doctor about the potential benefits of a magnesium supplement.

- ## **Vitamin D: The Sunshine Vitamin**

Vitamin D is essential for calcium absorption and bone health, but it also plays a role in muscle function. Studies have shown a link between vitamin D deficiency and pelvic floor dysfunction. Get your daily dose of vitamin D through sunlight exposure (in moderation), fortified foods, or supplements.

- ## **Supplements: A Helping Hand**

While a balanced diet is the foundation of pelvic health, certain supplements may offer additional support. Discuss the potential benefits of vitamin D, magnesium, or collagen supplements with your healthcare provider to see if they are right for you.

Remember, a healthy pelvic floor is a reflection of your overall health and well-being. By nourishing your body with a balanced diet rich in essential nutrients, you're not only supporting your pelvic floor but also investing in your long-term health and vitality.

## HOLISTIC HABITS: INTEGRATING MIND-BODY PRACTICES FOR OPTIMAL WELL-BEING

Your pelvic health isn't just about muscles and exercises; it's deeply interconnected with your overall well-being. In fact, research shows that stress, anxiety, and tension can negatively impact your pelvic floor, leading to tightness, pain, and even dysfunction. That's why it's crucial to embrace a holistic approach to pelvic health, one that nurtures both your body and your mind.

Mind-body practices, such as yoga, meditation, and stress management techniques, offer a powerful complement to your pelvic floor exercises. These practices not only promote relaxation and reduce stress but also cultivate body awareness, improve posture, and enhance your connection to your pelvic floor muscles.

- **Yoga: A Gentle Flow for Pelvic Floor Harmony**

Yoga, with its gentle movements and focus on breath, can be a wonderful way to strengthen and stretch your pelvic floor muscles. Certain poses, like Cat-Cow, Happy Baby, and Bridge Pose, gently engage and release the pelvic floor, promoting flexibility and improving blood flow. Additionally, yoga's emphasis on mindfulness and body awareness can help you tune into subtle sensations in your pelvic region, allowing you to better understand and control your muscles.

- **Meditation: Finding Calm and Centeredness**

Meditation, a practice of focused attention and awareness, can help reduce stress and anxiety, which are known contributors to pelvic floor tension. By calming your mind and cultivating a sense of inner peace, you create a more relaxed environment for your pelvic floor muscles to function optimally. Even a few minutes of daily meditation can make a significant difference in your overall well-being and pelvic health.

- **Stress Management Techniques: Tools for Resilience**

Chronic stress can wreak havoc on your body, including your pelvic floor. That's why it's important to develop healthy coping mechanisms to manage stress effectively. Deep breathing exercises, progressive muscle relaxation, and mindfulness practices can all help to reduce stress hormones and promote relaxation. Think about adding these methods to your regular practice, particularly when you're under a lot of stress.

- **The Mind-Body Connection: A Holistic Approach**

The body and mind are closely intertwined; they are not separate entities. What affects one affects the other. By cultivating a healthy mind-body connection, you can create a positive feedback loop that benefits your pelvic floor and overall health. When you're relaxed and stress-free, your pelvic floor muscles are more likely to function optimally. And when your pelvic floor is strong and healthy, you'll feel more confident, empowered, and at ease in your body.

In addition to yoga, meditation, and stress management techniques, there are many other mind-body practices that can support your pelvic health. Tai chi, qigong, and even simple walking in nature can all promote relaxation, mindfulness, and body awareness.

Remember, the key is to find practices that resonate with you and that you can incorporate into your daily life. By prioritizing your mental and emotional well-being, you're not only improving your pelvic health but also enhancing your overall quality of life.

# CHAPTER SEVEN

## EXPERT ADVICE AND PERSONALIZED SOLUTIONS

### WHEN TO SEEK HELP: RECOGNIZING SIGNS AND SYMPTOMS THAT WARRANT PROFESSIONAL GUIDANCE

Your body has an incredible ability to communicate with you, and it's essential to listen to its signals. When it comes to pelvic health, paying attention to subtle changes and seeking professional guidance when needed can make a world of difference. While pelvic floor exercises can be a powerful tool for strengthening and maintaining your pelvic health, there are times when seeking expert advice is crucial.

Remember, your pelvic floor is a dynamic and complex system, and sometimes, issues may arise that require a more personalized and targeted approach. If you experience any of the following signs or symptoms, it's important to consult with your healthcare provider:

- **Urinary Incontinence**

If you experience frequent or sudden urges to urinate, leakage when you cough, sneeze, or laugh, or difficulty emptying your bladder completely, it's essential to seek evaluation. These could be signs of stress incontinence, urge incontinence, or other bladder issues that require medical attention.

- **Bowel Problems**

Changes in bowel habits, such as constipation, fecal incontinence, or difficulty controlling bowel movements, should not be ignored. These issues can sometimes be related to pelvic floor dysfunction and may require further assessment.

- **Pelvic Pain or Pressure**

Persistent pain or a feeling of heaviness in your pelvic area can be a sign of pelvic organ prolapse, where one or more pelvic organs descend from their normal position. It's essential to address this issue promptly to prevent further complications.

- **Painful Intercourse**

If you experience pain during or after intercourse, it could be a sign of pelvic floor muscle tightness or other underlying issues. Seeking professional guidance can help identify the cause and find appropriate solutions.

- **Changes in Sexual Function**

If you notice a decrease in sexual desire, difficulty achieving orgasm, or changes in vaginal lubrication, it's worth discussing these concerns with your healthcare provider. Pelvic floor dysfunction can sometimes contribute to these issues, and appropriate treatment can often improve sexual function.

- **Persistent Back Pain**

While back pain can have various causes, it can sometimes be related to pelvic floor weakness. If you're experiencing persistent back pain, especially in the lower back, a thorough evaluation can help determine if pelvic floor dysfunction is a contributing factor.

## • **Difficulty with Pelvic Floor Exercises**

If you're having trouble identifying or engaging your pelvic floor muscles, or if you experience pain during exercises, seeking guidance from a pelvic floor therapist or other healthcare professional can be invaluable. They can provide personalized instruction, modifications, and alternative exercises to ensure you're practicing safely and effectively.

Remember, these are just a few examples of signs and symptoms that may warrant professional attention. Don't hesitate to reach out to your healthcare provider if you have any concerns about your pelvic health, even if they seem minor. Early intervention and appropriate treatment can often prevent further complications and improve your quality of life.

Your healthcare provider can conduct a thorough evaluation, including a physical exam, medical history review, and possibly additional tests, to determine the underlying cause of your symptoms and recommend the best course of action. This may involve pelvic floor physical therapy, medication, lifestyle changes, or other interventions.

By being proactive about your pelvic health and seeking professional guidance when needed, you're taking an important step towards a healthier, happier, and more fulfilling life.

## EXPLORING TREATMENT OPTIONS AND FINDING THE RIGHT FIT FOR YOU

When it comes to pelvic floor dysfunction, the good news is that you have options. A range of effective treatments exists, each tailored to address specific needs and preferences. Let's explore some of the most common approaches and how you can find the right fit for your unique situation.

- **Pelvic Floor Physical Therapy: Your Personalized Guide**

Think of a pelvic floor physical therapist as your personal trainer for your pelvic muscles. These specialized therapists are experts in assessing and treating pelvic floor dysfunction. They can teach you proper exercise techniques, provide manual therapy to release muscle tension, and offer guidance on lifestyle modifications.

Pelvic floor physical therapy is often the first line of treatment for many women, as it's non-invasive, effective, and personalized to your specific needs. It's particularly beneficial for those with stress incontinence, urge incontinence, pelvic organ prolapse, and pelvic pain.

- **Biofeedback: Seeing Your Progress in Real Time**

Sensors are used in the biofeedback technique to assess muscle activity. In the context of pelvic floor therapy, it allows you to see and hear how your muscles are contracting and relaxing. This visual and auditory feedback can help you learn to control your pelvic floor muscles more effectively.

Biofeedback is often used in conjunction with pelvic floor exercises to enhance their effectiveness. It can be particularly helpful for those who have difficulty isolating and contracting their pelvic floor muscles.

- **Medication: Targeted Relief for Specific Symptoms**

In some cases, medication may be recommended to manage specific symptoms of pelvic floor dysfunction. For example, anticholinergic medications can help reduce bladder overactivity and urge incontinence. Topical estrogen may be prescribed to improve vaginal tissue tone and elasticity, which can be helpful for women experiencing vaginal dryness or atrophy.

It's important to note that medication is not a cure for pelvic floor dysfunction, but it can provide relief from certain symptoms while you work on strengthening your pelvic floor muscles through exercise and other therapies.

- **Surgery: A Last Resort for Severe Cases**

Surgery is typically reserved for severe cases of pelvic floor dysfunction, such as pelvic organ prolapse that doesn't respond to conservative treatment. Various surgical procedures can repair or reinforce weakened muscles and ligaments, restore organ support, and alleviate symptoms.

While surgery can be effective, it's important to discuss the potential risks and benefits with your healthcare provider and explore all other options before considering this route.

- **Choosing the Right Approach: Your Personalized Path**

The best treatment for pelvic floor dysfunction depends on your individual needs, preferences, and the severity of your symptoms. A collaborative approach with your healthcare provider is crucial.

They can help you assess your options, consider your medical history and lifestyle factors, and develop a personalized treatment plan that aligns with your goals and values.

Remember, you are not alone in this journey. Many women experience pelvic floor issues, and a variety of effective treatments are available to help you regain control, comfort, and confidence.

By seeking professional guidance and exploring the options available, you can find the right path to a healthier and happier you.

# CHAPTER 8

## CELEBRATING YOUR STRENGTH: EMBRACING A CONFIDENT, VIBRANT FUTURE

### REAL-LIFE TRANSFORMATIONS THROUGH PELVIC FLOOR FITNESS

Stories have the power to inspire, motivate, and remind us that we are not alone in our struggles. As you embark on your own journey to pelvic floor fitness, let's draw inspiration from the real-life experiences of women who have overcome similar challenges and transformed their lives.

Meet Mary, a 68-year-old retired librarian who had been quietly battling urinary incontinence for years. She was hesitant to talk about it, feeling embarrassed and ashamed. But after reading about pelvic floor exercises, she decided to give them a try. To her surprise, she noticed a significant improvement in her bladder control within a few weeks. She no longer had to worry about leaks or accidents, and she felt more confident and empowered in her daily life.

"I can't believe how much these simple exercises have changed my life," Mary shared. "I feel like I've regained my freedom and independence. I can go out with friends, travel, and do the things I love without worrying about my bladder."

Then there's Sarah, a 72-year-old grandmother who had been experiencing pelvic pain and discomfort for years. Having tried various treatments, yet nothing seemed to work. After consulting with a pelvic floor therapist, she learned that weak pelvic floor muscles were contributing to her pain. Through a combination of targeted exercises, stretching, and lifestyle changes, Sarah gradually regained strength and flexibility in her pelvic floor. The pain subsided, and she was finally able to enjoy activities like gardening and playing with her grandchildren without discomfort.

"I'm so grateful for the information and support I received," Sarah said. "I never thought I would be able to live pain-free again. Now, I can enjoy life to the fullest and do the things that matter most to me."

Linda, a 65-year-old yoga enthusiast, discovered the benefits of pelvic floor fitness after experiencing a mild prolapse. She had always been active, but she realized that she had neglected her pelvic floor muscles. By incorporating specific yoga poses and pelvic floor exercises into her routine, she was able to strengthen her muscles and manage her prolapse without surgery.

"Yoga has not only helped me physically but also mentally and emotionally," Linda explained. "It's given me a greater sense of body awareness and connection to my pelvic floor. I feel stronger, more confident, and more empowered in my own body."

These are just a few examples of the many inspiring stories of women who have transformed their lives through pelvic floor fitness. Their journeys remind us that it's never too late to take charge of our health and well-being. Whether you're dealing with incontinence, pelvic pain, prolapse, or simply want to enhance your overall pelvic health, there are solutions available to help you achieve your goals.

By incorporating pelvic floor exercises into your daily routine, making healthy lifestyle choices, and seeking professional guidance when needed, you can overcome challenges, regain control, and embrace a life of confidence, comfort, and vitality. Remember, your story is still being written. With dedication, perseverance, and the right support, you too can achieve your pelvic floor fitness goals and enjoy a vibrant, fulfilling life.

## A LIFETIME OF VITALITY: YOUR ROADMAP TO CONTINUED PELVIC HEALTH AND WELL-BEING

As we reach the end of this empowering journey together, let's recap the essential tools and knowledge you've gained to nurture your pelvic health and well-being for years to come. Remember, the journey to a strong pelvic floor isn't a sprint; it's a lifelong marathon. By embracing consistent practice and healthy habits, you can maintain your progress and enjoy the benefits of pelvic floor fitness for years to come.

First and foremost, make pelvic floor exercises a non-negotiable part of your daily routine. Just like brushing your teeth or taking your vitamins, these exercises should become a habit that you prioritize. Whether it's a few minutes of Kegels while you're waiting in line or incorporating pelvic floor engagement into your daily walk, find ways to integrate these practices into your life seamlessly.

Variety is the spice of life, and it's also essential for maintaining a well-rounded pelvic floor fitness routine. Don't be afraid to experiment with different exercises, such as quick flicks, the elevator, or reverse Kegels, to keep your muscles challenged and engaged.

Remember, your pelvic floor isn't isolated; it's part of a larger system. Therefore, a holistic approach to pelvic health is crucial. Pay attention to your overall fitness level, maintain a healthy weight, and nourish your body with a balanced diet rich in fiber, protein, and essential nutrients.

Beyond exercise, there are other lifestyle habits that can significantly impact your pelvic health. Practice good posture, avoid heavy lifting whenever possible, and manage stress through relaxation techniques like meditation or deep breathing exercises.

Stay hydrated by drinking plenty of water throughout the day, and address any constipation issues promptly, as straining during bowel movements can weaken your pelvic floor muscles.

Don't give up if you run into obstacles or setbacks along the route. Remember, progress isn't always linear. It's OK that some days will be simpler than others. The key is to listen to your body, be patient with yourself, and celebrate your achievements, no matter how small they may seem.

Remember that you are not and never alone on this journey, YES. If you have any questions or concerns, don't hesitate to reach out to a pelvic floor therapist or other healthcare provider. They can offer personalized guidance, support, and additional resources to help you achieve your goals.

As you continue to prioritize your pelvic health, remember that it's an investment in your overall well-being. A strong pelvic floor can enhance your physical function, boost your confidence, and improve your quality of life. You'll be able to enjoy activities you love, whether it's dancing, gardening, or spending time with loved ones, without worrying about leaks, discomfort, or embarrassment.

So, keep practicing, keep learning, and keep celebrating your progress. Your pelvic floor fitness journey is an empowering one, and it can lead to a lifetime of vitality, confidence, and joy.

# CONCLUSION

For your pelvic floor fitness, remember that the journey you've embarked upon is a celebration of your strength, resilience, and unwavering commitment to your well-being. You've unmasked the unspoken, delved into the intricacies of your pelvic floor, and discovered the power of simple yet transformative exercises.

You've learned that pelvic health is not just about preventing leaks or managing discomfort; it's about embracing a life of confidence, vitality, and joy. It's about feeling empowered in your body, enjoying activities without worry, and experiencing a renewed sense of freedom and intimacy.

The knowledge you've gained is a treasure to be cherished and shared. Spread the word, empower other women, and break the silence surrounding pelvic health. By sharing your journey and encouraging others to prioritize their well-being, you create a ripple effect of positive change that extends far beyond yourself.

Remember, this book is just the beginning. Your journey to pelvic floor fitness is an ongoing process, a commitment to nurturing your body and honoring its wisdom. Embrace the tools and techniques you've learned, adapt them to your unique needs, and continue to explore new ways to enhance your pelvic health.

When in doubt, don't be reluctant to consult medical experts. Pelvic floor therapists, doctors, and other specialists can provide personalized support, answer your questions, and help you navigate any challenges that may arise.

As you go, bear the following important insights in mind:

- **Consistency is key**

Make pelvic floor exercises a regular part of your routine, just like brushing your teeth or taking your vitamins.

- **Listen to your body**

Pay attention to your body's signals and adjust your exercises as needed. If you are in pain or uncomfortable, get help from a specialist.

- **Embrace a holistic approach**

Nourish your body with a balanced diet, manage stress through relaxation techniques, and stay active to support your overall well-being.

- **Celebrate your progress**

Acknowledge and celebrate your achievements, no matter how small they may seem. It's clear from your journey that you are resilient and strong.

Remember, you are not alone. Millions of women are on this journey with you, seeking to improve their pelvic health and quality of life. Together, we can break down barriers, shatter stigmas, and empower women to take charge of their well-being.

So, go forth with confidence, knowing that you have the knowledge and tools to maintain a healthy pelvic floor for years to come. Embrace the vitality, embrace the joy, and embrace a life filled with comfort, confidence, and endless possibilities.

# BONUS

Surprise!

As a special thank you for choosing this book, I've included a bonus just for you. Scan the QR code below to unlock exclusive access to enhance your pelvic floor fitness journey. Also, I would like your honest and positive reviews on this book so as to know how helpful it was to you. This will be so much appreciated, Thank You.

Your journey to a stronger, healthier you doesn't end with this book. This bonus content is designed to provide you with ongoing support, motivation, and inspiration as you continue to prioritize your pelvic health and well-being.

# DEDICATION

To my extraordinary colleagues,

This book is a testament to the power of collaboration, support, and shared vision. It wouldn't exist without your unwavering belief in this project, your insightful feedback, and your tireless efforts to bring it to life.

Your expertise, passion, and dedication have been instrumental in shaping this book into a valuable resource for senior women seeking to reclaim their pelvic health and well-being. Your willingness to share your knowledge, offer guidance, and lend a helping hand has been truly inspiring.

This dedication is a heartfelt thank you for your invaluable contributions. May this book serve as a reminder of our shared commitment to empowering women, promoting health, and making a positive impact on the lives of others.

With deep gratitude and admiration,

[CHRISTIE JOSEPH]

www.ingramcontent.com/pod-product-compliance
Lightning Source LLC
Chambersburg PA
CBHW050824250726
48653CB00006B/2407